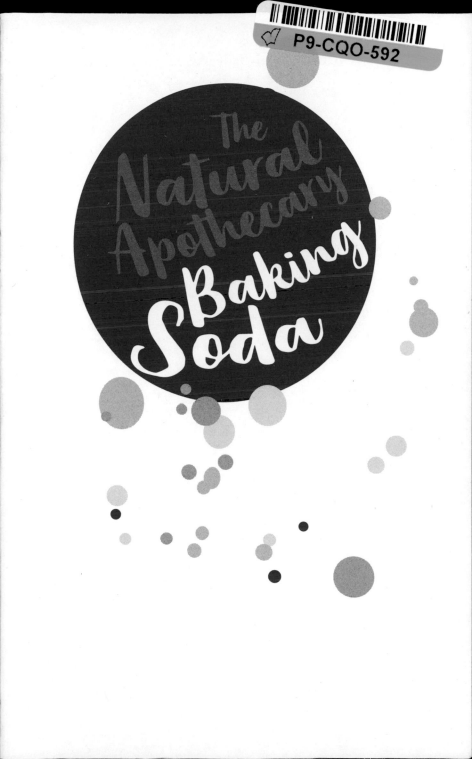

The Natural Apothecary

Baking Soda

Other titles in the Natural Apothecary series include:

The Natural Apothecary: Lemons
The Natural Apothecary: Cider Vinegar

About the author: Dr Penny Stanway practised for several years as a GP and child-health doctor before becoming increasingly fascinated by researching and writing about healthy diets and other natural approaches to health and wellbeing. Penny has written more than 20 books on health, food and the connections between the two. She lives with her husband on a houseboat in the Thames.

This edition published in the UK and USA 2019 by
Nourish, an imprint of Watkins Media Limited
89–93 Shepperton Road, London N1 3DF
enquiries@nourishbooks.com

1 3 5 7 9 10 8 6 4 2

Managing Editor: Daniel Hurst
Editor: Amy Christian
Head of Design: Georgina Hewitt
Typeset by: Integra Software Services Pvt. Ltd, Pondicherry
Production: Uzma Taj

Printed and bound in Great Britain by TJ International Ltd.

A CIP record for this book is available from the British Library

ISBN: 978-1-848993-68-6

www.nourishbooks.com

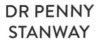

DR PENNY
STANWAY

The
Natural
Apothecary
Baking
Soda

USES FOR HOME, HEALTH
AND BEAUTY

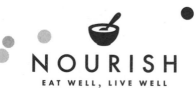

NOURISH
EAT WELL, LIVE WELL

CONTENTS

INTRODUCTION

For thousands of years, people have been using natural products to soothe, treat, beautify and cleanse. Herbs and spices, vegetables, fruits, nuts and berries have been mixed together to create traditional remedies that have been passed down through the generations. Many of these ingredients are still used in commercial products today, although are now often combined with harsh chemicals.

Today, we are used to relying on pharmacies and supermarkets, where there are hundreds of available products, each with a different purpose. We apply creams and ointments for various aches and pains, take vitamin supplements, and spend a fortune on lotions and potions for our skin, nails and hair. The number of cleaning products that are now on offer can be quite overwhelming!

By going back to basics, and taking a more natural approach to how we treat our diets, health, beauty regimes and household management, we are taking back control of what we are putting into our bodies and what we are exposing our families to.

Often used in cooking as a rising agent, baking soda (bicarbonate of soda) is also extremely valuable to us around the home, for our health and for beauty and hygiene purposes. It is very cheap to buy and can be found in any grocery store. It has been used by people all over the world in some form or other for generations.

What is baking soda?

Baking soda (bicarbonate of soda) is a white crystalline mineral powder with a multitude of uses, both domestic and commercial. This important mineral is available in small quantities as baking soda (bicarbonate of soda) from supermarkets and grocery stores and as 'sodium bicarbonate' from pharmacies (drugstores). You can also buy it in bulk online.

It is present (along with sodium carbonate) in the mineral known as Natron, which is deposited from salt lakes in various countries. Baking soda can also be mined as deposits of nahcolite in rock, and it is present in the water flowing from many hot springs. Today, though, it is mostly produced in factories, mainly by a method that mixes salt (sodium chloride), ammonia, calcium carbonate and carbon dioxide in water. A total of over 1 million tons is produced this way each year in various countries, including the USA, Italy, Egypt and China. The ancient Egyptians used Natron, which contains baking soda (bicarbonate of soda), but later on scientists were able

---

The benefits of Natron were known to the ancient Egyptians. They used it as part of their mummification rituals, as it absorbs water and prevents the growth of bacteria. Mixed with oil, it worked in the same way as soap, and was used for cleaning, as well as an antiseptic and an insecticide.

---

to separate the minerals that make up Natron to produce elements with more specific applications.

In the eighteenth century, The French Academy of Sciences had offered a prize to anyone who could come up with a way of producing sodium carbonate, known as soda ash, from common salt (sodium chloride). Sodium carbonate was in great demand as a multi-purpose detergent. Chemist Nicolas Leblanc won the contest, and set up a factory producing soda ash on a large scale.

Later on, in the 1830s, American bakers John Dwight and Austin Church were able to develop a process that enabled them to obtain baking soda (bicarbonate of soda) from soda ash. They manufactured and sold their baking soda to home bakers across the United States. Austin Church later founded the company Arm & Hammer with his two sons, now one of the largest global manufacturers of baking soda (bicarbonate of soda).

Baking soda (bicarbonate of soda) is also known as:

- baking soda (common in the US)
- bicarbonate of soda (common in the UK)
- 'bicarb'
- bread soda
- cooking soda
- sodium bicarbonate
- saleratus (a 19th-century term meaning 'aerated salt')

Our body's own internally produced sodium bicarbonate (as it is known by nutritionists and doctors) is a vital part of the acid–alkali balancing systems that keep us healthy. And by eating an alkali-producing diet (see pages 13–21) and, perhaps, taking sodium bicarbonate or applying it to our skin, we can help to treat certain common ailments (see pages 45-57).

It is definitely worth having baking soda to hand in the bathroom cabinet – as well as being advantageous to your health, it can be incorporated into your beauty regime, too. For example, it has a mildly abrasive nature, making it a great natural exfoliant. It can also be used to make toothpaste and 'bath bombs' and to coat dental floss. For more uses, see pages 60–71.

Baking soda is mildly alkaline in water but is also amphoteric, which means it can react with both acids and alkalis. It is useful in many commercial and domestic situations. It is used, for example, as a cake-raising agent, as well as to make baking powder, self-raising (self-rising) flour, soaps, domestic cleaning and deodorizing products, medications, water-softeners, 'dry' fire extinguishers and pesticides. It is incredibly useful for many household chores and can help keep your home fresh, clean and sparkling. For environmentally-friendly, non-toxic ideas for using baking soda as a natural cleaning product, see pages 73–107.

The names of certain other chemicals could sound confusingly similar to those unfamiliar with chemistry. These include:

- baking powder (which contains other ingredients besides sodium bicarbonate)
- sodium chloride (salt)
- washing soda (sodium carbonate or soda ash) and
- caustic soda (sodium hydroxide).

It is vital never to confuse any of these with sodium bicarbonate, so be sure that any container of white powder is clearly labelled.

CHAPTER ONE

BAKING SODA AND THE ACID-ALKALI BALANCE

1

BAKING SODA AND THE ACID-ALKALI BALANCE

You can treat yourself with baking soda (bicarbonate of soda) in three different ways. The first is by changing to an alkali-producing diet, of which full details are given on page 15. Changing to an alkali-producing diet is the most important starting point for treating nearly all the common ailments in the following chapter. Two other methods are taking baking soda (bicarbonate of soda) by mouth (see page 24), or applying it to the skin as a paste or in a bath (see pages 46–7).

Good health relies on our blood and other body fluids having the right acid–alkali balance. The bicarbonate that is naturally present in our body helps this to happen. The building blocks of our body's bicarbonate originate from food and drink.

As our cells produce energy from sugar (which is mainly derived from dietary carbohydrate), they release carbon dioxide. This can react reversibly with water to form carbonic acid – a weak acid that breaks down reversibly into bicarbonate and hydrogen.

Many foods contain carbonates or other organic substances that the body can convert into bicarbonate. ('Organic' is used here in its chemical sense, meaning these substances contain only carbon, oxygen and, perhaps, hydrogen.)

Any bicarbonate consumed in food or drink neutralizes a certain amount of stomach acid; any excess is absorbed from the intestine into the blood.

Some people also get bicarbonate from antacids or other medications.

Fluid accounts for nearly 60 per cent of the weight of a man's body and 55 per cent of a woman's. The average man's body, weighing 70kg/154lb, contains 42 litres/74 pints/89 US pints.

Acid–alkali balance

Each body fluid is a watery solution containing electrolytes (substances that can break down into electrically charged particles called ions). A fluid is said to be acidic if its concentration of hydrogen ions is greater than that of its hydroxyl ions, and alkaline if the other way around.

One hydrogen ion and one hydroxide ion can combine to form a molecule of water. A solution is neutral (neither acidic nor alkaline) if its hydrogen and hydroxide-ion concentrations are equal.

What is pH and why is it important?
A body fluid's pH ('potential of Hydrogen') represents its hydrogen-ion concentration, which in turn indicates its acid–alkali balance. Each number on the pH scale represents a ten-fold decrease in hydrogen-ion

concentration from the one below and a ten-fold increase from the one above.

A fluid becomes more acidic as its hydrogen-ion concentration rises and its pH falls, and becomes more alkaline as its hydrogen-ion concentration falls and its pH rises.

The pH scale goes from 0 to 14, with 7 neutral for water. Because pH is temperature-dependent, a neutral pH for blood at body temperature would be 6.7. But we would die if it were neutral! It must always be alkaline. And it must stay within a very small range of pH.

The pH of body fluids

Most body fluids are alkaline. Their pHs are regulated by our lungs, kidneys and buffers (see pages 10–11). And they affect each other in various important ways.

- Normal arterial blood and tissue fluid have an average alkaline pH of 7.4 (range 7.35–7.45). Venous blood is slightly less alkaline at 7.36 (since cells produce acids, releasing hydrogen ions that can enter veins).
- Intracellular fluid has a pH of about 7.
- Pancreatic juice is particularly alkaline at pH 7.5–8.8. Urine can be acidic or alkaline (pH 4.5–7.5). Stomach juice is very acidic (pH 1–2). As stomach contents enter the duodenum (the first part of the small intestine), they are alkalinized by bile and pancreatic juice. The skin's surface moisture, from skin oil and sweat, mostly has a pH of 4.5–5.75, but is slightly less acidic in the armpits and around the genitals.

Does a change in pH matter?

A change in the pHs of blood, tissue fluid or intracellular

fluid can have vitally important consequences to our health, wellbeing and even life itself, by affecting:

- Energy production (measurable as a person's 'basal metabolic rate')
- Molecular reactivity
- Bonding of oxygen and carbon dioxide to haemoglobin (the pigment in red blood cells) and therefore the transport of oxygen to cells and carbon dioxide from cells
- Oxidation (a low pH encourages the production of 'free radicals' – also known as reactive oxygen-containing ions)
- Muscle-cell contraction
- Enzyme activity
- 'Folding', and therefore function, of proteins (including structural ones)
- Exchange of potassium and sodium across cell membranes
- Bio-electric signalling in and between cells
- Calcium balance
- Fatty acid and cholesterol metabolism
- Levels and activity of, and sensitivity to, certain hormones (for example, adrenaline, thyroxine and growth hormone)
- Cell growth, differentiation, multiplication and apoptosis ('cell suicide')
- Cell mobility
- Behaviour of red blood cells (a low pH makes them stack up so that they cannot properly transport oxygen, carbon dioxide, nutrients and waste products)

- Size and behaviour of white cells (a low pH makes them smaller and less active)

The degree of pH change required to affect cells isn't always clear. However, a very abnormal pH (below 6.8 or above 7.8) makes the normal folded shape of each protein molecule begin to 'unravel'. If this continues, life continues for only a few hours.

How the body responds to changes in pH
When the body-fluids' normal pHs are threatened or actually changed by diet, lifestyle, disease or medication, the following things happen:

- Lungs exhale more carbon dioxide to reduce acidity, or less to increase acidity.
- Kidneys excrete more inorganic acidic anions (mainly chloride) to reduce acidity, or fewer to increase acidity. This pH-regulation is slower than that of the lungs.
- Body fluids buffer (minimize) pH changes by changing the levels of bicarbonate, non-volatile weak inorganic acidic ions or acids.
- Liver can metabolize organic acidic anions (for example, it converts lactate into glycogen).
- Cell membranes allow a greater or smaller passage of various ions between cells, tissue fluid and blood.
- Sympathetic nervous system produces more or less adrenaline to stimulate the heart, lungs and kidneys.
- Sweat contains more or fewer acidic anions (such as phosphates, sulphates, chlorides and lactates).
- The above responses affect the following indepe

pH-regulating factors in body fluids:

1 Strong-ion difference. Most body fluids are alkaline because their concentration of strong alkaline cations (sodium, potassium and, to a lesser extent, calcium and magnesium) is greater than that of strong acidic anions (chloride, sulphate, phosphate, lactate). The strong-ion difference and, therefore, the pH, fall with a decrease in strong cations or an increase in strong anions, and vice versa. The strong-ion difference is affected by our diet and the activity of our digestive tract, kidneys and cells.

2 Carbon dioxide. This flows from cells to tissue fluid to blood. It can also flow the other way. The amount in our body fluids varies with changes in metabolism, circulation and breathing rate.

3 Non-volatile weak inorganic acids.

Changes in the above factors in turn change our bicarbonate and hydrogen-ion levels.

Bicarbonate and the lungs

ᵇᵒn dioxide produced by cell metabolism is carried in the
ᵉ lungs, where any excess is breathed out to prevent
ᵇlood pH (and so making it less alkaline).
ᵗens to lower our blood pH, we
ᵉ rapidly and exhale more carbon

kidneys

ᵃte from the blood and excrete

about 20 per cent of it. If something threatens to lower our blood pH, the kidneys excrete less bicarbonate, and vice versa.

Bicarbonate buffer

Buffers change their concentration to help maintain the body's acid–alkali balance. Bicarbonate is our most important buffer. Bicarbonate ions can raise pH (thereby increasing alkalinity) by joining with hydrogen ions to form carbonic acid.

ACIDOSIS AND ALKALOSIS

Acidosis is a 'push' towards acidity, or, more accurately (because blood, tissue fluid and intracellular fluid are never actually acidic), a push towards lowered alkalinity. This is associated with the accumulation of acid and hydrogen ions, or loss of bicarbonate.

The lungs, kidneys and buffers try to compensate so as to maintain or restore a normal blood pH. While this is perfectly normal, if prolonged or extreme it can 'strain' the body and cause symptoms. Depending on the success of compensation, the blood pH either remains within its normal range or falls below 7.35 (which causes symptoms).

Alkalosis is a 'push' towards over-alkalinity. The lungs, kidneys and buffers try to compensate for this. Depending on their success, the blood pH may remain within its normal range or rise above 7.45. Alkalosis is much less common than acidosis.

11

Carbonic acid can lower pH (thereby reducing alkalinity) by breaking down into hydrogen and bicarbonate ions. Carbonic acid is such a weak acid that in itself it has negligible acidity.

Does mild acidosis cause symptoms?

Researchers claim that almost all adults eating a typical Western diet have mild ongoing acidosis. The question is whether this 'chronic low-grade metabolic acidosis' can cause symptoms. Experts have long contested the idea, but we now know it can happen.

Whether such symptoms result from the lungs, kidneys and buffers compensating for the threat to the normal range of pH, or from a slight reduction in pH that nevertheless remains within the normal range, is unclear.

What causes mild acidosis?

It seems sensible to assume that any cause of metabolic acidosis with a pH below 7.35 could, if less severe, cause mild metabolic acidosis. But researchers think the two main causes of mild metabolic acidosis are:

- An acid-forming diet
- An age-related decline in kidney function.

We cannot prevent ageing, but we can adjust our diet (see page 13). We can also deal with conditions that can cause more severe metabolic acidosis and might therefore cause the mild type. Finally, we can consider taking an alkali supplement (see page 38).

Balancing your diet

An acid-producing diet is the norm in the Western world. Such a diet lacks enough alkali-producing vegetables and fruit to balance the intake of acid-producing meat, fish, eggs and cereal-grain food, and the result is chronic low-grade metabolic acidosis. Bicarbonate plays an important part in the regulating systems that help our body counter acidosis.

Acidic foods

An acidic food is not the same as an acid-producing food. Acidic foods taste acidic because they contain organic food acids (such as citric, acetic, oxalic, malic, pyruvic and acetylsalicylic acids), 'organic' here meaning that they contain only carbon, oxygen and hydrogen. Some acidic foods, such as citrus fruit, vinegar, yoghurt, soured (sour) cream, buttermilk and soured milk, actually taste acidic. Others, such as beer, cider (apple cider), honey, treacle (molasses), maple syrup, coffee, and 'natural' cocoa and chocolate (dark unsweetened varieties made from cocoa beans that haven't been 'Dutch-processed') are acidic but don't taste so.

Organic food acids don't produce acid in the body because the liver breaks them down into carbon dioxide and water. Excess carbon dioxide is exhaled and excess water is eliminated by the kidneys and lungs. So most acidic foods have virtually no effect on our acid–alkali balance; a few, including lemon juice and cider vinegar (apple cider vinegar), even have an alkali-producing effect.

Acid-producing foods

These foods are not acidic and do not taste acidic, but when digested and metabolized produce acids that make body fluids less alkaline. An acid-producing diet is rich in meat, grain and sugar and carbonated drinks and low in vegetables and fruit.

Certain acid-producing foods produce acid by releasing more strong acidic anions (such as sulphate/sulfate, which can join with hydrogen ions to form sulphuric acid) than strong alkaline cations (see page 63), such as potassium, which can join with bicarbonate to form potassium bicarbonate.

The kidneys can eliminate only a limited load of strong acidic ions each hour, so any surplus causes acidosis.

Acid-producing foods include:

- Protein (such as in meat, fish, eggs, cheese, beans)
- Grain foods (such as bread, breakfast cereal, pasta, cakes, biscuits, many puddings, and rice; note that refined-grain foods are more acid-producing than wholegrain foods)
- Sugar (especially refined sugar – both white and brown).
- Certain acid-producing foods and food constituents have an acidifying effect that is independent of the diet's total acid-producing load:
- Table salt (sodium chloride) encourages acidosis by decreasing the blood's strong-ion difference. (It does this by increasing chloride more than sodium and encouraging the kidneys to excrete potassium.)
- Tea, coffee, cocoa, chocolate and pulses and legumes (such as soya beans and chickpeas) contain purines that are metabolized to uric acid.
- Alcohol encourages acidosis by increasing lactate production.

Foods that cause an 'acid tummy'

Strongly acidic foods (such as lemon juice), plus certain acid-producing foods and drinks, can stimulate the production of enough stomach acid to cause 'acid indigestion'. Such foods include those made from white sugar or white flour; tea, coffee (even decaffeinated) and cocoa; and beer and wine (possibly because of protein-breakdown products such as amino acids and amines produced during fermentation).

Alkali-producing foods

These foods contain more strong alkaline than strong acidic ions, so when metabolized, they produce alkaline salts such as bicarbonate. They include:

- vegetables and fruit
- certain nuts, beans, grains, cheeses and sugars.

Many experts assert that alkali-producing foods should compose 80 per cent of our diet, with acid-producing foods making up the rest. However, the average Western diet is composed mainly of acid-producing foods, with vegetables and fruit (the major alkali-producing foods) contributing only 2 per cent!

Our diet

The effect of our overall diet on our acid–alkali balance is more important than the effects of individual foods. This is because, when a meal has been digested and metabolized, its net effect is either acidic or alkaline.

Our aim should be to eat an alkali-producing diet. We can deal with temporary acidosis from an occasional acid-producing meal, but weeks or months of chronic low-grade acidosis may cause symptoms.

Research suggests the two key factors affecting our acid–alkali balance are our intake of:

- protein (especially meat), which is acidifying, and
- potassium (most importantly, from vegetables and fruits), which is alkalinizing.

Protein
Animal protein is found in meat, fish, eggs and dairy food. Research suggests that dairy food's high calcium levels help to protect against any acidosis-promoting effect of its protein. Vegetable protein is found mainly in beans and peas and in nuts, grains and other seeds.

Potassium
Potassium is plentiful in vegetables and fruits and produces strong alkalizing ions in body fluids. Particularly rich sources include green leafy vegetables, tomatoes, bananas, dates and avocados.

What are acid-producing and alkali-producing foods and drinks?
Burning a food in a laboratory produces heat and reduces the food to acidic or alkaline ash. This is the equivalent of our cells burning food to produce energy. So measuring the pH of a burnt food's ash indicates the acid- or alkali-producing effect of that food in our body. The ash produced by the

THE ACID-PRODUCING POTENTIAL OF VARIOUS FOODS

'High', 'Medium' and 'Low' refer to a food's acid-producing potential. Most of us could do with eating less 'high' acid-producing food:

Meat and fish	High:	Pork, beef, shellfish
	Medium:	Eggs, lamb, sea fish, chicken
	Low:	Freshwater fish
Dairy foods	High:	Hard cheese, ice cream
	Medium:	Soft cheese, cream
	Low:	Yoghurt, cottage cheese, milk
Grain-foods	High:	White flour, white bread, white pasta
	Medium:	Wholemeal and wholegrain bread; biscuits, white rice, corn, oats
	Low:	Brown rice, sprouted-wheat (Essene) bread, spelt flour and bread
Nuts	Medium:	Pistachios, peanuts, cashews, walnuts
	Low:	Macadamias, hazelnuts
Fats and oils	Low:	Margarine, sunflower oil, corn oil, butter
Sugar, honey,	Medium:	Chocolate, white sugar, brown sugar
confectionery	Low:	Processed honey, treacle (molasses)

Condiments	High:	Most vinegar, soy sauce, salt
	Medium:	Mustard, mayonnaise, tomato ketchup.
Drinks	High:	Spirits, beer, soft drinks
	Medium:	Coffee, wine, fruit juice
	Low:	Tea
Vegetables	Medium:	Potatoes without skins; pinto, navy and lima beans
	Low:	Kidney beans
Fruits	Medium:	Cranberries
	Low:	Plums, prunes
Other	Low:	Coconut milk

THE ALKALI-PRODUCING POTENTIAL OF VARIOUS FOODS

'High', 'Medium' and 'Low' refer to a food's alkali-producing potential. Most of us could do with eating or drinking more of these foods:

Fruits	Medium:	Avocado, tomato, lemon, dried figs, rhubarb
	Low:	Pineapple, raisins, dried dates, strawberries, grapefruit, apricot, blackberries, orange, peach, raspberries, banana, grapes, pear, blueberries, apple, coconut

Vegetables	High:	Cucumber, sprouted seeds
	Medium:	Radishes, celery, garlic, spinach, beetroot (beet), French beans, carrots, chives, turnips
	Low:	Watercress, leeks, courgettes (zucchini), peas, cabbage, cauliflower, mushrooms, swede (rutabaga), onion, lettuce, potatoes with skins, asparagus, Brussels sprouts, sweet potatoes
Beans	Medium:	White ('navy') beans, fresh (or frozen) soya beans (soybeans)
	Low:	Tofu, soya flour, lentils
Dairy food	Low:	Goat's cheese, goat's milk, soya milk, buttermilk
Grains	Low:	Buckwheat, spelt, wild rice, quinoa
Nuts and seeds	Low:	Almonds, Brazil nuts, chestnuts, pumpkin seeds, sunflower seeds, flaxseeds, sesame seeds
Oils	Medium:	Olive oil, flaxseed oil
	Low:	Rapeseed oil (canola), olive oil
Sugar, honey	High:	Raw honey, raw sugar
	Medium:	Maple syrup
Drinks	High:	Herb tea, lemon water
	Medium:	Green tea
	Low:	Ginger tea
Other	Low:	Cider vinegar (apple cider vinegar)

average vegetarian diet is significantly more alkaline that that from the average omnivorous diet. This is mainly because animal protein has a high acid-producing potential.

How to improve your diet

If you have been eating a typical Western diet, help to rebalance it by using the above lists as a guide to favouring alkali-producing foods. An added bonus is that the vegetable and fruit content of such a diet provides a wealth of health-enhancing factors, including vitamins, phenolic compounds, carotenoids, plant hormones, salicylates, fibre and omega-3 fats.

- As already noted, research shows that the two factors that best predict acidosis are too much protein (especially too much red meat) and not enough potassium (mainly from vegetables and fruit). However, although the matter is still being studied, my understanding is that a lack of vegetables and fruit is the most likely cause of health problems from a typical Western diet.
- Eat at least five servings a day of vegetables and fruit, of which three should be vegetables, two fruit. Potatoes (and yams, cassava and plantain) are important for an alkali-producing diet as they are potassium-rich. However, they don't count towards your five-a-day as they are classed not as vegetables but as starchy carbohydrates (like bread, rice, noodles, pasta and sweetcorn). Peas, beans and lentils count as only one helping a day, no matter how much you eat, because they contain fewer nutrients than do other vegetables. However, sweet potatoes, parsnips, swedes and turnips do count towards your five-a-day.

Fruit and vegetable juices count as only one helping a day, however much you drink.

- Five-a-day is officially recommended in the US and many other countries. But one 2007 US study found that only 32 per cent of people met the guidelines for vegetables, only 28 per cent for fruits, and fewer than 11 per cent for vegetables and fruit. Also, one in four ate no vegetables on a daily basis and three in five ate no whole fruits!
- Some experts recommend up to nine helpings of vegetables a day, as well as two of fruit. This would certainly decrease your appetite for acid-producing foods!
- Cook vegetables lightly and use the potassium-rich cooking water in soups or gravy, or eat them raw.
- Include alkali-producing food in every meal and snack.
- Keep a food diary of everything you consume over seven days. Highlight acid-producing foods in red, alkali-producing in green. This will help you to evaluate the balance of your diet.
- Use the Diet Plate, or the Eatwell Plate, developed by the food standards agency in the UK.
- Avoid added salt, use less, or choose potassium-enriched 'low' salt.

Adding baking soda to your diet

Baking soda (bicarbonate of soda) is most commonly found in kitchens. One reason for this is that when combined with water and acid, it creates tiny carbon-dioxide bubbles that aerate (raise or leaven) dough, batter or cake mix, making it puffier and lighter. Yeast and eggs were the main raising agents until the late 1700s, when scientists found that baking soda (bicarbonate of soda) acted faster.

Baking soda (bicarbonate of soda) can be inexpensively purchased in supermarkets, grocery stores, hardware stores and chemists. It is very likely that you already have some in your kitchen cupboard. You may prefer to source larger quantities online, as the boxes sold for home cooks are often quite small. Baking soda can be used:

- on its own, if the recipe contains an acidic food or cream of tartar (a powder that produces acid when mixed with water)
- in baking powder
- in self-raising (self-rising) flour.

Baking soda in cooking

Baking soda (bicarbonate of soda) softens dried beans and peas before they are used in such dishes as fried mung beans. In combination with water and an acidic ingredient, it produces bubbles that puff up starchy ingredients such as wheat, polenta (also known as cornmeal or maize meal) or chickpea flour (also known as gram flour, garbanzo flour and besan).

It is also an important ingredient of falafels, which are particularly popular in North Africa and the Middle East.

Baking soda (bicarbonate of soda) and baking powder come into their own when making sweet treats such as apple fritters, honeycomb and sweet waffles.

Almost every cake recipe contains baking soda (bicarbonate of soda) either as the sole raising agent or in baking powder.

Tips for using

Do

- Store in an airtight container in a cool dry place.
- Sift with other dry ingredients several times before using to ensure thorough mixing.
- Mix ingredients rapidly and cook a mixture without delay to prevent carbon-dioxide bubbles that were released during mixing in the bowl from escaping.
- Use the amount recommended in a recipe. Too little can make a cake rise poorly and the finished product tough and dense. Too much can produce super-size bubbles that make a bread or cake rise too rapidly, which produces a coarse, open-textured loaf or cake and makes fruit and nuts sink. Also, the bursting bubbles make a cake sink in the middle.
- If cooking at high altitude, use less than a recipe suggests, as carbon-dioxide bubbles expand faster when air pressure is relatively low.
- Make chicken skin crispy by rubbing with baking soda (bicarbonate of soda) before cooking.
- If a sauce or casserole tastes too acidic, stir in ½–1 teaspoon of baking soda (bicarbonate of soda).
- Soak dried beans in water containing baking soda (bicarbonate of soda). This makes them cook faster, reduces their content of starch and complex carbohydrates, which could ferment in the gut and produce gas, and makes them more digestible. Use 1 teaspoon of baking soda (bicarbonate of soda) for each 200g/7oz/1 cup beans. Soak in a large saucepan of water for 12–24 hours, then rinse and cook.
- Check whether old baking soda (bicarbonate of soda) is usable by mixing ¼ teaspoon with 2 teaspoons of vinegar – it should bubble at once.

Don't

- Add it to green vegetables to retain their colour as they boil, because its alkalinity destroys vitamin C (ascorbic acid).
- Be tempted to use too much, as it could react with fat or oil to form traces of soap, giving the finished product a strange after-taste!
- Substitute it with baking powder, as baking soda (bicarbonate of soda) has four times the raising power.

Taking sodium bicarbonate
Sodium bicarbonate is available from supermarkets and groceries as 'bicarbonate of soda' in the UK and 'baking soda' in the US. It is not the same as 'baking powder' (see page XII).

Dose
One teaspoon of the powder contains 600mg of baking soda (bicarbonate of soda). The usual adult dose, taken 1–4 times a day, is:

Under-60s:	½–1 teaspoon
Over-60s:	¼–½ teaspoon

In the UK, baking soda (bicarbonate of soda) is also available from pharmacies as 500mg capsules and 600mg tablets. In the US, it is available as 325mg and 650mg tablets.

The US Food and Drug Administration (FDA) sets the maximum dose at 16g per day for the under-60s; 8g per day for the over-60s.

For optimal absorption into the blood, take baking soda (bicarbonate of soda) on an empty stomach. For acid indigestion, take it when you have discomfort. Doctors

TIPS AND WARNINGS

- Don't take baking soda (bicarbonate of soda) daily for more than 2 weeks without consulting a doctor.
- Don't confuse it with baking powder.
- Unless agreed with your doctor, don't take it if you're on a sodium-restricted diet or have high blood pressure, kidney, lung, heart or liver disease, fluid retention, urination problems, low blood calcium or anal bleeding.
- Take only small doses if pregnant, breastfeeding or over 60.
- Consult your doctor first if you are on prescription drugs, as some interact with baking soda (bicarbonate of soda). Some of those that do interact include benzodiazepines, calcium- or citrate-containing preparations, ephedrine, fluoroquinolones, iron, ketoconazole, lithium, methenamine, oral anti-diabetes drugs, quinidine, steroids, tetracycline and urine-acidifying medications.
- Check with a doctor or sports coach if considering taking baking soda (bicarbonate of soda) to enhance your exercise performance.
- Don't give baking soda (bicarbonate of soda) to a child unless discussed with a doctor and the dose agreed.

sometimes give baking soda (bicarbonate of soda) in an intravenous (IV) 'drip'.

As baking soda (bicarbonate of soda) neutralizes stomach acid, it releases carbon dioxide, which causes belching. Any excess baking soda (bicarbonate of soda) passes into the intestine and, when absorbed into the blood, has an alkalinizing effect.

Side effects
Depending on the dose and the person, baking soda (bicarbonate of soda) can cause:

- **Metabolic alkalosis**, with nausea, vomiting, numbness, tingling, tremor, muscle twitching, cramp, dizziness, fainting, confusion
- High blood sodium, possibly with thirst, ankle swelling, high blood pressure, frequent urination, seizures, **heart failure** or even a stroke
- Low blood potassium, possibly with weakness, fatigue, cramp, tingling, numbness, **nausea, vomiting**, bloating, **constipation**, irregular heartbeat, large amounts of urine, thirst, confusion, hallucinations or fainting
- Nervous-system depression, possibly with headache, drowsiness, nausea, vomiting, lack of coordination, dizziness or confusion
- Milk-alkali syndrome – abnormally high blood calcium in people with poor kidney function, if baking soda (bicarbonate of soda) is taken with dairy products, **calcium supplements** or calcium-containing antacids. If continued, this can cause calcium deposits, **kidney stones** and **kidney failure**
- Allergic swelling of the face, lips, tongue and throat,

and difficulty in breathing. This needs urgent medical attention.

If you suspect a serious reaction, or have taken an overdose, call a doctor or an ambulance; in the US, call the National Poison Control Center on 1-800-222-1222. If you go to a doctor or hospital, you or someone else should bring the container of baking soda (bicarbonate of soda).

Benefits of an alkali-producing diet
Changing to an alkali-producing diet is the most important starting point for the home treatment of many common ailments. Natural remedies using baking soda (bicarbonate of soda) can be found on pages 43-57, and while these may offer short-term solutions to some health problems, it is worth understanding the longer-term effects that our diet has on some chronic conditions.

NOTE
Major dietary changes should always be made in consultation with a doctor.

Anxiety
Anxiety can encourage either acidosis or alkalosis. In addition, acidosis can encourage anxiety. One way in which anxiety can cause acidosis is by increasing the stress hormone adrenaline. This tenses muscles, which in turn boosts energy production in muscle-cells, releasing an acidic anion called lactate.

Conversely, some anxious people breathe rapidly, so they exhale too much carbon dioxide, encouraging respiratory alkalosis.

As for acidosis encouraging anxiety, people on a high-protein diet have acidosis and are allegedly more likely to feel irritable. Also, chronic acidosis encourages anxiety by encouraging magnesium loss from bones.

Arthritis

Rheumatoid arthritis is linked with the intake of meat, wheat, sugar, salt and coffee – all of which are acid-producing.

Other research indicates a lower likelihood in Mediterranean countries, where the traditional diet contains little red meat. Rheumatoid arthritis is also less common in vegetarians and vegans who, in turn, are less likely than meat-eaters to have an acid-forming diet. And it's less common in people who eat more cruciferous vegetables (such as cabbage and broccoli) and fruit.

People with rheumatoid arthritis are more likely to have antibodies to milk, cereal, eggs, fish and pork. Food sensitivity is encouraged by an acid-producing diet. So it's possible that such a diet might encourage rheumatoid symptoms as part of an immune response triggered by a food sensitivity (see 'Food allergy', page 33). All this suggests that an acid-forming diet encourages rheumatoid arthritis.

Osteoarthritis can be linked with acidosis. The kidneys normally excrete acidic salts, but if they can't do this fast enough, such salts can crystallize in joint fluid and trigger inflammation.

Gout causes arthritis and can be triggered by acidosis (see page 48).

Asthma

Food allergy triggered by an acid-producing diet can be responsible for asthma (see 'Food allergy', pages 33). Pre-existing acidosis also makes airway-widening medication less effective early in an attack.

Airway tightening during an attack triggers deep rapid breathing. Too much carbon dioxide is then exhaled, leading to respiratory alkalosis. This triggers the bicarbonate buffering system to normalize the alkalosis. But if a person's diet is acid-producing, they could be short of bicarbonate, in which case their alkalosis might continue or even worsen.

Sodium bicarbonate can relax airways and encourage them to respond to airway-widening medication.

Cancer

Early research increasingly supports the idea that acidosis can encourage cancer. For example, studies indicate that cancer cells sometimes stop multiplying when the pH is relatively alkaline (just above 7.4). This pH also encourages more oxygen to enter cancer cells – which is good because low oxygen encourages cancer cells to multiply. Other research shows that cancer cells engender acidosis around them, which makes weak-alkali anti-cancer drugs less effective.

Several links suggest that acidosis encourages cancer:

- Obesity is associated with more bowel, gallbladder, kidney and prostate cancers. Researchers also speculate that acidosis encourages obesity. So acidosis may prove to be an underlying factor behind both obesity and cancer.
- A high protein intake encourages bowel and prostate cancer, whereas eating plenty of vegetables discourages bowel, breast and stomach cancer. Similarly, an acid-

producing diet encourages acidosis. So acidosis may
prove to encourage certain cancers.
• Studies suggest that acidosis encourages diabetes. People
with diabetes have an increased risk of certain cancers
(for example, liver and pancreas cancer). So acidosis may
prove to encourage both diabetes and cancer.

Unproven treatment claims include:

• Applying baking soda (bicarbonate of soda) paste to a rodent
ulcer (basal-cell carcinoma) or squamous-cell skin cancer.
• Taking ascorbic acid and baking soda (bicarbonate of
soda) for stomach or bowel cancer. These release sodium
ascorbate and the hope is that this will damage cancer
cells.
• Taking baking soda (bicarbonate of soda) mixed with
maple syrup.

Finally, bicarbonate is proving useful in diagnosing cancer
and monitoring treatment. This is because cancer cells
convert bicarbonate to carbon dioxide, and magnetic
resonance imaging (MRI) scans can monitor changing
carbon-dioxide levels.

Cataracts
These could be linked with acidosis as they can result from
ageing or stress encouraging a build-up in the eyes' lenses
of insoluble calcium salts of phosphoric or uric acid. Taking
baking soda (bicarbonate of soda) helps to dissolve these
salts, as does a potassium-rich diet.

Convulsions

Convulsions occur in 70–80 per cent of people with epilepsy, despite their medication, and acidosis may be a factor.

Convulsions can also result from a slow-onset immune reaction caused by a food sensitivity enabled by acidosis (see 'Food allergy', page 33).

Depression

Depression is sometimes reported as a side-effect of a high-protein, low-carbohydrate diet, which in turn is associated with low-grade metabolic acidosis.

Depression can also result from a slow-onset immune reaction caused by a food sensitivity enabled by acidosis (see 'Food allergy', page 33).

Diabetes, pre-diabetes and metabolic syndrome

Researchers believe that acidosis encourages cells to become resistant to insulin. Normally, this hormone enables blood sugar to enter cells. But if cells are resistant, blood-sugar rises. The pancreas then produces extra insulin to prevent high blood sugar. This 'pre-diabetes' can have adverse effects, including obesity, fluid retention, high blood pressure, raised LDL-cholesterol, fatigue, faintness, mood swings, dry skin, skin tags and darkened skin.

Some people with pre-diabetes have a collection of problems together called the metabolic syndrome. This greatly encourages diabetes, heart disease and strokes and is characterized by having three of the following: insulin resistance, excess fat around the waist, high blood pressure, high blood fats, or low HDL-cholesterol (the helpful sort).

Dieters may develop acidosis if their diet contains insufficient vegetables and fruit. This is a particular problem because many people with pre-diabetes, metabolic syndrome or diabetes are overweight and repeatedly trying to slim.

Before oral anti-diabetic drugs, and insulin, doctors often treated diabetes with baking soda (bicarbonate of soda).

Fatigue and poor concentration

These can result from metabolic acidosis. One possible reason is exhaustion from rapid breathing triggered as the body tries to correct a low pH.

A second possible cause is a slimming diet, particularly if low in carbohydrate. This leads to a shortage of sugar for energy production and means cells must use protein or fat as an energy source instead. But converting these nutrients to usable fuels takes longer than converting carbohydrate to sugar. This is a particular disadvantage for brain cells, hence the fatigue and poor concentration. What's more, burning fat for energy produces acidic ketones. Not only can the resulting acidosis cause fatigue but it also encourages pre-diabetes, which can trigger tiredness. The lack of sugar also affects heart muscle (see 'Heart disease', page 35), causing low energy.

A third possible reason is a slow-onset immune reaction associated with a food sensitivity enabled by acidosis (see 'Food allergy', page 33).

Fibromyalgia

With this condition you have stiff, weak, knotted shoulder and back muscles and tender points on hips, knees, neck, spine, elbows or buttocks. There may also

FOOD ALLERGY

Chronic low-grade metabolic acidosis is associated with low bicarbonate in the body. This means pancreatic juice may not contain enough bicarbonate to alkalinize acidic food residues entering the duodenum. As a result, its enzymes may not break down proteins properly; also, acidic food residues can damage the intestinal lining. Whole undigested protein molecules can then pass through the 'leaky' lining into the blood and sensitize the immune system.

When someone sensitized to a protein next eats it, one of two things can happen. The first is that immunoglobuin E (IgE) antibodies can adhere to it in the intestine, blood or elsewhere, forming tiny particles called immune complexes, which can cause trouble (for example, by blocking tiny blood vessels). The second is that white cells can release inflammatory substances (such as histamine and leucotrienes), which can increase the production of potentially damaging free radicals (reactive oxygen-containing ions).

Food-allergic symptoms beginning within minutes or up to 2 hours are caused by a fast-action immune response. This can result from eating even only a little of the particular food. Common culprits are milk, eggs, peanuts, tree nuts, fish, shellfish, soya, wheat and oranges. Possible symptoms include swollen face, lips, mouth, tongue and throat; vomiting; **diarrhoea**; abdominal pain; itching; allergic rhinitis ('hayfever'); urticaria (hives or 'nettle-rash'); asthma; and conjunctivitis. Pre-existing eczema may worsen. At worst there is anaphylactic shock (with potentially fatal breathing difficulty, a fall in blood pressure and, perhaps, loss of consciousness).

Food-allergic symptoms beginning later, though within 72 hours, are caused by a slow-onset immune response. Affected people may react to several foods. Possible symptoms include flushing, nausea, vomiting, diarrhoea, oesophagitis (inflamed gullet), gastritis (inflamed stomach), abdominal pain, fatigue, muscle weakness, aching and stiffness, eczema, joint pains, palpitation, fluid retention (perhaps with bloating, headaches, fluctuating weight, temporarily raised blood pressure, depression, convulsions and restless legs) and gallstones.

be fatigue, poor sleep, headaches, dizziness, numbness, tingling, irritable bowel and bladder, restless legs, poor memory and concentration, depression, anxiety, over-sensitivity to noise, light and temperature, and Raynaud's phenomenon.

Many experts blame metabolic acidosis, suggesting that this deposits acidic ions in muscles and connective tissue. Various studies support this idea.

Heart disease

The findings below indicate that acidosis encourages low energy, an irregular heartbeat (atrial fibrillation), chest pain on exercise (angina), heart attacks and heart failure. Whether chronic low-grade metabolic acidosis (as with a typical Western diet) has similar effects isn't yet known. Many studies show that acidosis can:

- Reduce energy production from sugar in heart-muscle cells; energy production from fats and proteins takes longer than from sugar, so low energy is an early problem.
- Irritate the coronary arteries (if the pH is below 7.35), encouraging tiny tears. LDL-cholesterol then seeps into the artery lining and attracts white blood cells. These white cells provoke inflammation, which oxidizes cholesterol. They then engulf the oxidized cholesterol. Calcium infiltrates the damaged artery walls, while smooth-muscle cells produce collagen to cover the leaks. All this causes atherosclerosis – stiffening of the arteries plus narrowing by a chalky, fatty, fibrous, white-cell-laden substance called atheroma building up in the artery walls. Patches of atheroma can rupture, encouraging a blood clot, which could trigger a heart attack.
- Interfere with the passage of potassium, sodium and calcium across cell membranes, and also rob the body of potassium, calcium and magnesium as they neutralize acids in the urine. This weakens heart-muscle, prevents the normal conduction of electrical messages, and makes sodium and calcium accumulate in blood, encouraging high blood pressure and atheroma.
- Increase LDL-cholesterol (the sort that's potentially

dangerous if oxidized) and decrease HDL-cholesterol (the protective sort).
- Increase adrenaline, which speeds the heart and boosts its cells' need for oxygen.
- Encourage insulin-resistance; blood sugar then can't enter cells normally, so rises, triggering extra insulin production. But high insulin has adverse effects, such as boosting LDL-cholesterol.
- Raise fibrinogen, encouraging blood clots, which can block a coronary artery.

Blood pH is lowest (at its most acidotic) during sleep, which is when fatal heart attacks are most common.

Palpitation can result from a slow-onset immune reaction associated with a food sensitivity enabled by acidosis (see 'Food allergy', page 35).

High blood pressure
Acidosis seems to encourage high blood pressure. The probable culprit is a lack of vegetables and fruit, since there is no evidence that a high protein intake in itself raises blood pressure. Taking baking soda (bicarbonate of soda) (or any other alkalizer) may reduce blood pressure. Acidosis makes cells more resistant to insulin. The pancreas then produces extra insulin to prevent high blood sugar. This makes arteries over-sensitive to adrenaline, thereby encouraging high blood pressure.

Infertility
To be successful, a sperm must first undergo a process called capacitation – the alteration of the surface of its head

so it can adhere to an egg. This is done by fertilization-promoting peptide, a substance produced by the prostate and mixed with sperm on ejaculation.

Capacitation occurs in the cervix or womb but occurs only if the alkalinity is right. This happens just before ovulation, when cervical glands produce 'sperm-friendly' mucus that is suitably alkaline, abundant, clear, elastic and watery, and contains strands that are aligned to encourage sperm penetration.

Osteoporosis

Osteoporotic bone is light and fracture-prone. The risk factors include age; too much or too little exercise; smoking; too little bright outdoor light; a lack of dietary calcium, magnesium, zinc, vitamins C, D and K, plant hormones or fibre; too much 'diet cola' (because of its phosphoric acid); early menopause; anorexia; and various medications and illnesses (including gut and thyroid disorders – some of which can result from acidosis).

Studies also implicate inflammation, which can result from acidosis.

Acidosis also impairs bone health by decreasing the activity of bone-building cells (osteoblasts) but increasing the activity of bone-destroying cells (osteoclasts).

Research suggests that acidosis may draw calcium from the bones to partner acidic anions in the urine.

Finally, researchers believe chronic low-grade metabolic acidosis from an acid-producing diet can be a factor. In particular, they point to a lack of vegetables and fruit.

Vegetables and fruit contain many 'bone-friendly' nutrients and have an alkali-producing effect.

Several studies suggest an alkaline supplement could have a similarly helpful alkalinizing effect.

Overweight and obesity

Acidosis encourages resistance to the hormone insulin. Normally, insulin enables blood sugar to enter cells. But if cells are resistant, blood sugar rises and the pancreas produces extra insulin to convert surplus sugar into fat.

Many conditions are encouraged by, or associated with, both obesity and acidosis. For example, obesity and acidosis each encourage heart disease, high blood pressure, strokes, diabetes, metabolic syndrome, heartburn, gallstones, pancreatitis, osteoarthritis, gout, kidney stones, asthma, fatigue, depression, sleep apnoea ('stop-breathing' attacks during sleep), underactive thyroid, absent periods, infertility and certain cancers (though any influence from acidosis is only suggested as yet).

Since acidosis also encourages obesity, it is tempting to speculate that this is a linking factor.

It would also be worth investigating whether acidosis is responsible for other conditions encouraged by obesity – including age-related macular degeneration (an eye disease), Alzheimer's disease, deep vein thrombosis, pulmonary embolism, pre-eclampsia (a pregnancy condition), high blood fats, polycystic ovary syndrome and liver disease.

People who don't eat meat – and are therefore less likely to have chronic low-grade metabolic acidosis – are also less likely to be obese.

Another fact is that most obese people are malnourished. Severe malnutrition decreases the bicarbonate content of pancreatic juice, encouraging acidosis.

If you want to lose weight, be aware that for the same calorie intake you can eat an amazingly larger amount of vegetables and fruit than of foods rich in fat, protein and carbohydrate. For example, you could swap one 250g/9oz fat- and sugar-free muffin for 900g/2lb pineapple, half a melon, 2 pears, 150g/5oz grapes, half a kiwi, half a papaya and 2 wholemeal rolls! Or 200g of cashew nuts for 8 baked jacket potatoes.

Avoid a high-protein, low-carbohydrate diet, as this encourages acidosis. An added bonus of an alkali-producing diet is that you can eat more yet still lose weight, because eating more vegetables and fruit can turn a fat-storing tendency into a fat-burning one.

Poor circulation

Research strongly suggests that acidosis encourages the narrowing and stiffening of arteries known as atherosclerosis (see 'Heart disease', page 35). Although the body compensates for the obstruction to normal circulation by developing high blood pressure, atherosclerosis is eventually likely to reduce the rate of the blood supply. This, in turn, can strain the normal working of all the body's cells. Some of the most obvious of the many possible symptoms are:

- Abnormal sensitivity to cold
- Impotence in men
- Lack of libido
- Paleness
- Poor memory
- Slow wound healing (especially on legs, ankles and feet).

Premature ageing

Scientists have long searched for lifestyle factors that encourage a long life and discourage age-related conditions such as wrinkles, age spots, arthritis, heart disease, diabetes, cancer, osteoporosis, age-related macular degeneration, cataracts, poor memory and Alzheimer's.

Long-lived peoples include certain groups in Russia (the Georgians), Pakistan (the Hunzas), Ecuador, China, Tibet and Peru. One link is that they tend to live at high altitudes and drink mountain water rich in alkaline minerals such as calcium, which help prevent acidosis. Another is their consumption of fermented vegetables, fruit, milk, cereal grains, meat or fish. These contain acids (such as lactic, acetic and malic) produced during fermentation but metabolized to alkali in the body.

Another related fact is that spa water from medicinal springs is invariably alkaline.

It is sometimes suggested, though hasn't yet been proved or disproved, that chronic low-grade metabolic acidosis also encourages:

- Hyperactivity in children
- Lupus
- Multiple sclerosis
- Myasthenia gravis
- Pre-menstrual syndrome
- Sarcoidosis
- Schizophrenia
- Scleroderma

In contrast, chronic low-grade metabolic acidosis is very common in peoples eating a typical Western diet. And ageing exaggerates acidosis because declining kidney function reduces the excretion of excess acid:

The pH change accompanying acidosis has damaging effects on cells and metabolism in general (see page 35), some of which encourage premature ageing. For example, it is associated with structural changes in proteins, the oxidation of fats and a lower oxygen supply to cells.

Stroke

Just as acidosis can encourage coronary heart disease and heart attacks (see pages 35–6), so too can it encourage arterial disease and strokes ('brain attacks' caused by blood clots or bleeds from cerebral arteries) in the brain.

An acid-producing diet is a possible contributory factor.

CHAPTER TWO
NATURAL REMEDIES FOR HEALTH

2
NATURAL REMEDIES FOR HEALTH

Baking soda (bicarbonate of soda) is a long-standing natural remedy for many ailments and can play a significant part in good day-to-day health and hygiene. It is particularly useful for treating skin irritations and digestive issues.

Mixed with water, baking soda (bicarbonate of water) can be taken as a restorative drink, or applied directly to the skin as a paste. Add it to bath water either on its own or with relaxing essential oils for a soothing whole-body treatment.

For more general advice on including baking soda (bicarbonate of soda) as part of a longer-term diet and lifestyle regime, see pages 3-41.

How to make soda water
Drinking soda water is a pleasant way of taking baking soda (bicarbonate of soda). Make it with a 1-litre/35fl oz/4 cup rechargeable soda siphon, a disposable one-shot screw-in cartridge of pressurized carbon dioxide, plus baking soda (bicarbonate of soda) and water.

1 Add ¼–½ teaspoon of baking soda (bicarbonate of soda) to 1 litre/35fl oz/4 cups of water.
2 Put this into the soda siphon, then add the carbon dioxide.
3 Flavour it with plain syrup or fruit syrup if you like.

Unlike many soft drinks, soda water does not contain phosphoric acid, which encourages calcium loss from bones.

Alternatives to baking soda (bicarbonate of soda)
If you cannot take baking soda (bicarbonate of soda) for some reason, discuss with your doctor whether an alternative alkalinizer (such as potassium bicarbonate or calcium carbonate) would be appropriate.

Apply baking soda (bicarbonate of soda) to the skin

Baking soda (bicarbonate of soda) dissolved in water has an alkaline pH of 8.3 and can ease the itching, discomfort and inflammation of certain skin conditions. Two ways of applying it are making it into a paste or adding it to a bath.

Baking soda (bicarbonate of soda) paste

Put 1 tablespoon of baking soda (bicarbonate of soda) into a small bowl and stir in about 1 teaspoon of water. Apply a thin layer of the paste to the skin. Let the paste dry on the skin, then leave it on for 30 minutes before rinsing it off with water.

Alkaline bath

Add 100–200g/3½–7oz/½–1 cup of baking soda
(bicarbonate of soda) to a bath of comfortably hot water. Add
a few drops of lavender or other essential oil for fragrance.

TESTING URINE PH

Unusually acidic urine suggests that the kidneys are eliminating
excess acid. The most common reason for this is an acid-
forming diet.

The pH of normal urine ranges from 4.6 to 8.0. It's more
acidic in the morning than in the evening. If you test your
urine, it's best to test '24-hour' urine (all the urine passed in 24
hours and pooled in one container, or cupfuls collected each
time you urinate and pooled in one container). Urine pH test
strips are available from pharmacies or on the internet.

PLEASE NOTE

- The strategies outlined should not take the place of
  medical diagnosis and therapy.
- Consult a doctor about possible causes and treatments
  for continuing, worrying or worsening symptoms.
- You can help prevent and treat most ailments with a
  healthy diet, adequate hydration, regular exercise, daily
  outdoor light, effective stress management, a sensible
  alcohol intake and no smoking.

Digestion, diet and gut health

Diarrhoea
If persistent severe diarrhoea originates in the small intestine, it can cause metabolic acidosis from the loss of bicarbonate. If it originates in the large intestine it can cause metabolic alkalosis from the loss of chloride.

Diarrhoea can also result from a slow-onset immune reaction enabled by acidosis.

Heal from the inside out
Eat an alkali-producing diet (see pages 13–16).

Regular treatment
Consider taking oral rehydration salts (from a pharmacy) or ½ teaspoon of baking soda (bicarbonate of soda) in a glass of water up to four times a day.

Gout
Gout is associated with needle-like crystals of sodium urate (specifically, monosodium urate monohydrate) in joints or under the skin. Urates form when purines from food and from the body's cells are broken down by the body into uric acid, which is carried in the blood as urate. The kidneys normally excrete excess urate, but with acidosis they may not do so fast enough, so urate levels rise. Some people report that taking baking soda (bicarbonate of soda) alleviates or cures an attack. By reducing acidosis, this presumably (it is not yet proven) enables more sodium urate to dissolve in the blood, encouraging urate crystals in the joints to dissolve. Gout attacks are more likely at night, which is when the body is particularly acidic. In an online

poll of people with gout, 85 per cent said that baking soda (bicarbonate of soda) helped.

Heal from the inside out
Eat an alkali-producing diet (see pages 13–16).

Regular treatment
Consider taking ½ teaspoon of baking soda (bicarbonate of soda) four times a day for a week.

Indigestion, heartburn, gastritis and peptic ulcer
Acidosis from an acid-producing diet increases the stomach's production of bicarbonate *and* acid. The acid encourages 'acid' indigestion, heartburn, peptic ulcers and gastritis (inflamed stomach lining). When the stomach contents enter the duodenum, pancreatic juice provides bicarbonate to neutralize the acid. This stimulates stomach-lining cells to produce more bicarbonate; at the same time they automatically produce even more acid.

Taking baking soda (bicarbonate of soda) can neutralize excess acid. But its sodium is absorbed into the blood and some people are believed to be sodium-sensitive. So antacids such as calcium carbonate or magnesium or aluminium hydroxide are probably preferable (and scarcely absorbed).

Note that too little stomach acid can also cause indigestion.

To help identify poor stomach-acid production, drink a teaspoon of baking soda (bicarbonate of soda) in a glass of water on an empty stomach. If you don't belch within 5–10 minutes (from acid converting baking soda into carbon dioxide) you may have low acid, in which case antacids are unlikely to relieve indigestion.

Regular treatment
Consider taking ½–1½ teaspoons of baking soda (bicarbonate of soda) in a glass of water. Alternatively, take another antacid or discuss with your doctor or pharmacist whether to take an acid-suppressant.

Skin problems

Theoretically, at least, acidosis (see page 11) can trigger or worsen various skin conditions. This is because it encourages:

- Itching
- Inflammation
- Allergy
- Infection
- Raised insulin (see 'Diabetes', page 31–2), which encourages dry skin, and skin tags and dark skin on the neck, under the breasts and in the armpits and groin
- Pain from broken or inflamed skin.

One way of treating many skin conditions is to eat an alkali-producing diet to prevent acidosis.

Applying baking soda (bicarbonate of soda) directly to affected skin combats certain problems.

Allergic contact dermatitis
Reduce itching by applying a paste of baking soda (bicarbonate of soda) and water.

Cuts and grazes
Apply a paste of baking soda (bicarbonate of soda) and water to help cutas and grazes heal more quickly.

Eczema
Have an alkaline bath. Add 100–200g/3½–7oz/½–1 cup of baking soda (bicarbonate of soda) to a bath of comfortably hot water. Add a few drops of lavender or other essential oil for fragrance.

Fungal skin and nail infection (including athlete's foot)
Soak feet in a bowl of water containing a handful of baking soda (bicarbonate of soda) for 20 minutes daily.

Rub a paste of baking soda (bicarbonate of soda) and water into affected toenails or fingernails and leave it on for 20 minutes.

Sprinkle baking soda (bicarbonate of soda) between the toes each day.

Heat rash
Apply a paste of baking soda (bicarbonate of soda) and water.

Insect bites and stings
Apply a paste of baking soda (bicarbonate of soda) and water. (Wasp stings respond to something acidic, such as vinegar; remember: B for Bicarbonate and Bee stings, V for 'Vasp' stings and Vinegar.)

Itching
Apply a paste of baking soda (bicarbonate of soda) and water, or have a bicarbonate bath.

Nappy (diaper) rash
Sit the baby in a bicarbonate bath for a few minutes then pat dry.

Small burns, or sunburn
Apply a paste of baking soda (bicarbonate of soda) and cold water to help prevent blistering and scarring. The cold paste takes heat from burnt skin; also, baking soda (bicarbonate of soda) dissolves endothermically (removing heat from its surroundings as it dissolves), which absorbs further heat.

Splits on the ends of the fingers
Rub in a little baking soda (bicarbonate of soda) powder if the split is moist or make it into a paste first with a little water if it is dry.

Splinter
Apply a paste of baking soda (bicarbonate of soda) and water, cover with a sticking plaster (adhesive bandage) and leave overnight to help draw out the splinter.

Oral health

Dental care
Baking soda (bicarbonate of soda) cleans and brightens teeth. It also counteracts the acidity that is produced by mouth bacteria from traces of sugars and other refined carbohydrates, and which encourages tooth decay.

Regular treatments
Coat your toothbrush bristles with baking soda (bicarbonate of soda) before brushing your teeth. This 'dry-brushing' with bicarbonate removes plaque better than 'wet-brushing'.

Some people advocate making a fresher-tasting paste by mixing equal amounts of baking soda (bicarbonate of soda) and fine sea salt. Salt boosts the flow of saliva (which has anti-bacterial properties, so helping prevent tooth decay) and contains the alkaline mineral sodium, which helps to counteract acidity.

Make a cleansing, refreshing mouthwash by mixing ½ teaspoon baking soda (bicarbonate of soda) in ¼ glass of warm water. Take a mouthful and swish it around your mouth.

Make a whitening toothpaste by mixing baking soda (bicarbonate of soda) with 3 per cent hydrogen peroxide solution. Use it once a week and rinse your mouth thoroughly with water afterwards. Hydrogen peroxide is available online or from certain pharmacies (drugstores).

Tooth decay and gum disease
Mouth bacteria encourage tooth decay because they feed on food debris and produce acids that corrode tooth enamel. Bicarbonate inhibits the formation of plaque (a sticky layer of food debris that can develop into tartar, which in turn encourages gum disease) on teeth. It also neutralizes acids produced by bacteria, helps prevent tooth decay, and increases calcium uptake by enamel.

Regular treatment
Clean teeth with bicarbonate-containing toothpaste or baking soda (bicarbonate of soda).

Bad breath
An acid-forming diet encourages bad breath from residues of meat or refined carbohydrate on or between the teeth. Mouth bacteria can break these down and release unpleasant-smelling compounds.

Regular treatment
Rinse your mouth with ½ teaspoon of baking soda (bicarbonate of soda) in a glass of water.

Quick fix
For super fresh and minty breath, try dipping a piece of chewing gum into water and then sprinkling with baking soda (bicarbonate of soda). Chew on the gum for 5–10 minutes.

Mouth ulcers
Baking soda (bicarbonate of soda) can soothe ulcers and aid healing.

Regular treatment
Dissolve 1 teaspoon of baking soda (bicarbonate of soda) in a glass of water and swirl a mouthful around your mouth every 2–3 hours.

General health

Headache
Headaches are a possible symptom of metabolic acidosis with a pH below 7.35. It's also possible, though unproven, that chronic low-grade metabolic acidosis can cause

headaches as a result of the body's buffer systems working extra hard to keep the blood's acid–alkali balance within its normal tightly controlled range.

Heal from the inside out
Eat an alkali-producing diet.

Quick fix
If you eat an acid-producing diet or have other reason to believe you might have acidosis, consider taking ½–1 teaspoon of baking soda (bicarbonate of soda) in a glass of water to help cure a headache.

Muscle cramp
Acidosis can draw magnesium from the body to accompany acidic anions, such as lactate, in the urine, encouraging cramp. Rest as necessary to allow your blood to clear its acidic lactate.

Heal from the inside out
Eat an alkali-producing diet.

Regular treatment
Consider taking ½ teaspoon of baking soda (bicarbonate of soda) every 6 hours if you get repeated cramp.

Cystitis
A person with acidosis produces relatively acidic urine. This can inflame the bladder and encourage urine infections. The resulting cystitis causes painful, frequent urination. Alkalinizing the body with baking soda (bicarbonate of soda) helps to neutralize excess acid in the urine. It also kills bacteria and makes certain antibiotics more effective.

Regular treatment
Affected women should consider drinking ½ teaspoon of baking soda (bicarbonate of soda) in a glass of water four times a day. Other alkalinizing remedies are available from pharmacies.

NOTE

See a doctor if this is your first attack, or you are no better within 2–3 days. Men and children should always see a doctor.

General infections
It is suggested that increasing the blood's alkalinity helps to prevent or treat bacterial and viral infections.

Heal from the inside out
Eat an alkali-producing diet.

Regular treatment
If you suspect an infection, drink ½ teaspoon of baking soda (bicarbonate of soda) in a glass of water four times a day.

Hayfever or itchy eyes
Baking soda (bicarbonate of soda) can help to soothe irritated eyes.

Regular treatment
Bathe itchy eyes once or twice a day with an eyewash made from mixing 1/2 teaspoon baking soda (bicarbonate of soda) in ½ cup cold water. The solution will keep for 1–2 days in the refrigerator.

Cold or flu
Clear a blocked nose or sinuses with a baking soda (bicarbonate of soda) inhalation.

Quick fix
Add 1 teaspoon of baking soda (bicarbonate of soda) and 1 teaspoon of salt to a bowl of just-boiled water. Lean over the bowl, with your face near to the water and place a towel over your head, covering the bowl. Inhale the vapour for 20 minutes, or as long as necessary.

CHAPTER THREE

NATURAL
BEAUTY
TREATMENTS

3

NATURAL BEAUTY TREATMENTS

Baking soda (bicarbonate of soda) is a great beauty aid. It softens water, so you need less soap to wash your face and body and less shampoo to wash your hair. This is good because the more soap you use, the more you strip valuable natural oils and acidity from your skin and scalp.

The very mildly abrasive nature of baking soda (bicarbonate of soda) means that it helps to clean the skin. Its tiny rounded particles also have gentle exfoliating properties, helping to dislodge dead cells. This smoothes and brightens skin, making it look younger and healthier. What's more, it stimulates the skin's tiny blood vessels (capillaries), giving the skin a soft attractive glow. It can also help to clear blackheads.

When present in toothpaste, baking soda (bicarbonate of soda) can help to remove dental plaque (the sticky film of food residues and bacteria that accumulates on teeth) and tartar (hard, calcium-impregnated plaque that encourages gum disease). Its alkalinity is helpful for teeth, too. For example, it can neutralize the acidity released during the breakdown of sugars and other refined carbohydrates by mouth bacteria. This is important, because acidity encourages teeth to decay.

Baking soda (bicarbonate of soda)'s alkalinity has antiseptic and antifungal actions that can help to prevent or treat minor skin and scalp infections. It also has a deodorant action that is thought to result from neutralization of odoriferous short-chain fatty acids in the sweat produced in the armpits, for example.

Finally, baking soda (bicarbonate of soda) is a common ingredient in the effervescent balls of bath salts known as 'bath bombs'.

Here you'll find tips for using bicarbonate for personal care, as well as bicarbonate-containing recipes for toiletries such as toothpaste, deodorant and 'bath bombs'.

NOTE

- Baking soda can dry out or irritate the skin. Always test out treatments on a small patch of skin before using.
- Don't use baking soda on your skin more than twice a week.

Bathing

To soften bathwater add 100g/3½oz/½ cup baking soda (bicarbonate of soda) to your bath. A few drops of fragrant oil will make your bath-time particularly sybaritic. Cedarwood, frankincense and lavender essential oils are said to be relaxing, while geranium, jasmine, neroli and ylang ylang are considered uplifting, and cardamom stimulating and refreshing.

For extra cleaning power, so you don't need to use soap, add several squeezes of shampoo.

For a seaside-spa-style bath, add 100g/3½oz/½ cup baking soda (bicarbonate of soda) plus 100g/4oz/½ cup sea salt to the water.

To eliminate toxins, reduce bloating and prepare your body for a good night's sleep, add 100g/3½oz/½ cup baking soda (bicarbonate of soda) and 2 tablespoons Epsom salts to your evening bath water. Add a few drops of your chosen essential oil for ultimate relaxation.

Bath bombs

These are colourful fragrant lumps of bath salts that fizz when added to bath water. Next time you have a bath, put a 'bath bomb' in the water and watch it fizz as its citric acid and baking soda (bicarbonate of soda) react with the water to release bubbles of carbon dioxide. They also make lovely gifts – make a few in different colours and wrap them in tissue paper.

200g/14oz/2 cups baking soda (bicarbonate of soda)
200g/7oz/1 cup citric acid

10 drops fragrant essential oil of your choice
2–3 drops of food colouring
1 teaspoon almond oil or baby oil

1   Mix the baking soda (bicarbonate of soda) and citric acid together in a bowl

2   Add the essential oil and the food colouring and mix again.

3   Add the almond oil or baby oil, a few drops at a time, until the mixture is crumbly but just clumps together when firmly squeezed.

4   Firmly press the mixture into moulds – try plastic egg boxes, silicone or other non-stick fairy-cake moulds, little yoghurt pots, or special moulds from craft stores.

5   Leave the mixture to dry in the moulds for a week, before using.

CITRIC ACID

Citric acid is available from a pharmacy or online. This is one of the alpha hydroxy acids (AHAs) beloved of beauty-product manufacturers. Skin products containing AHAs have moisturizing and exfoliating properties, as they help the skin retain water and encourage the separation of dead skin cells..

Deodorizing

Adding baking soda (bicarbonate of soda) to your bath water (see 'Bathing', page 62) will help to keep you odour-free.

Alternatively, pat on baking soda (bicarbonate of soda) as a dry deodorant.

Sprinkle baking soda (bicarbonate of soda) between toes, or into tights (pantyhose) or socks, as an alternative to talcum powder to help keep feet fresh and dry.

Shake a little baking soda (bicarbonate of soda) on a new sanitary pad before use, to reduce odour.

Homemade deodorant

½ teaspoon of baking soda
   (bicarbonate of soda)

1–2 drops of water
1 drop of fragrant essential oil

1 Mix all the ingredients together in a small bowl.
2 To use, smooth a little of this deodorant paste under your
   arms.

Smooth skin

Exfoliating

After cleansing your skin, make an exfoliant paste by
mixing about 3 parts of baking soda (bicarbonate of soda)
to 1 part of water. Gently rub this into your skin, then
rinse off.

To smooth roughened lips, rub them with a paste made
by mixing baking soda (bicarbonate of soda) with lemon
juice. Rinse and then apply some lip balm.

Smooth cuticles by wetting them, rubbing in a little
baking soda (bicarbonate of soda), then rinsing, drying and
applying moisturizer.

Softening dry, rough or hard skin

Make a skin-softening paste by combining baking soda
(bicarbonate of soda) and extra-virgin olive oil. Add
fragrance, if you like, by adding a few drops of lavender,
rose or neroli essential oil. Smooth the paste over your
hands, elbows, the bottoms of your feet or other areas of dry,
rough or hard skin. Wait for 30 minutes then rinse off the
paste with warm water and immediately smooth in some
moisturizing cream.

Shaving

Mix baking soda (bicarbonate of soda) with water to form
a loose paste and apply this to your skin before shaving as
an alternative to soap lather or shaving cream or gel. This is
less 'drying' to the skin than most soaps because it doesn't
reduce the skin's natural oils and acidity.

Quickly soothe a shaving rash by smoothing on a paste made from baking soda (bicarbonate of soda) and water, as above. You can wash the paste off visible areas such as your face or legs before you see other people.

Help to prevent a shaving rash by smoothing on a paste made from baking soda (bicarbonate of soda) and water, as above.

Clearing blackheads

Twice a day, clean and dry your face. In a small bowl, mix 1 tablespoon of baking soda (bicarbonate of soda) with about 1 teaspoon of water to make a paste. Rub this over your skin to help loosen and remove blackheads, leave for 10–20 minutes, then rinse. Now help to restore your skin's natural acidity by patting on a little cider vinegar (apple cider vinegar).

Baking soda face mask

The natural exfoliating properties of baking soda (bicarbonate of soda) are combined here with two of nature's other beauty heroes: apple cider vinegar and lemon juice.

½ cup baking soda (bicarbonate of soda)

1 tablespoon apple cider vinegar
1 teaspoon lemon juice

1   Mix the ingredients together in a small bowl to form a paste.
2   Apply to clean skin in circular motions using your fingertips.
3   Sit for at least 10 minutes and then rinse off with warm water.

Hair care

Remove a build-up of products, such as hairsprays and hair gels, by squeezing your usual amount of shampoo into the palm of your hand and mixing in 1–2 teaspoons of baking soda (bicarbonate of soda). Use this to wash your hair, then rinse well. Repeat, then condition your hair.

Make your own dry shampoo and dry-clean greasy hair when short of time by sprinkling it with baking soda (bicarbonate of soda), rubbing this through with your hands, then brushing thoroughly. Add a few drops of essential oil to the baking soda for a pleasing scent.

Foot care

Soothe aching feet by adding 4 tablespoons of baking soda (bicarbonate of soda) to a washing-up bowl of warm water. Put this on the floor, sit on a chair and soak your feet for 10–15 minutes. Add several drops of essential oil for fragrance.

Hand and nail care

Make a paste from 1 tablespoon of baking soda (bicarbonate of soda) mixed with a little water. Exfoliate cuticles by rubbing the paste into the area around the finger nails with a nail brush. Rinse off with warm water.

Mix the juice of half a lemon with enough baking soda (bicarbonate of soda) to create a paste. Apply the paste to remove stains or discoloration from finger nails. Leave for 5 minutes then rinse off with warm water.

Cleaning brushes

Make up and hair products can build up on brushes, leaving an unpleasant residue. Fill a bowl with warm water water and add 2–3 tablespoons of baking soda (bicarbonate of soda). Soak the brushes for 15–20 minutes, then rinse and lay out on a clean towel to air dry.

Removing fake tan

Mix baking soda with lemon juice to create a paste and apply to any areas of uneven or patchy fake tan. Rub the paste off with a cloth before showering.

CHAPTER FOUR
NATURAL CLEANING PRODUCTS

4

NATURAL CLEANING PRODUCTS

Baking soda (bicarbonate of soda) is a non-toxic product that can help to keep your home and laundry fresh, clean and fragrant. It can help in many ways and in many places around the home. Making your own cleaning products may seem like a lot of work compared to buying them, but many of the suggestions in this chapter are extremely quick and easy, and use everyday ingredients that you will most likely find you already have in your storecupboard.

Making your own products is fun, and quite addictive. It will allow you to take control over your own environment, as well as saving you money. We all have busy lives, and it may seem easier to pick up a different brightly-coloured bottle for each of your household chores, but consider the benefits of leaving them behind in the store.

Greater control

Store-bought products often contain a cocktail of harsh chemicals which can be absorbed into the skin and breathed in. By making your own products you can be sure that only safe, natural ingredients are being used. You can also control the strength of the product by diluting as required, meaning that you can use the same product at different strengths for different tasks around the home.

More cost effective

Many of the ingredients used in natural cleaning products are easily available and inexpensive. The most commonly used ingredients are store-cupboard staples like lemons, vinegar and baking soda (bicarbonate of soda).

Environmentally friendly

The use of natural products is often referred to as 'green cleaning'. Making your own products cuts out the levels of pollution that are made during the production of commercial cleaning products, as well as reducing plastic consumption. Not all of the packaging for store-bought cleaning products is recyclable. Some commercial cleaning products may contain ingredients that are tested on animals.

Safer for pets and children

If you know that there are no 'nasties' in your cleaning products, you do not need to worry so much about other family members – especially pets and children – accidentally coming into contact with them. This also applies to any family members who might suffer from allergies – homemade natural products are unlikely to cause asthma attacks or irritation to the skin and eyes.

Create a nicer atmosphere

Homemade products that contain essential oils may have additional beneficial effects on your mood. Think of it as combining a deep cleaning session with an aromatheraphy treatment for the whole family!

Using baking soda in natural cleaning products

Baking soda (bicarbonate of soda) is mildly abrasive and has degreasing, water-softening and deodorizing qualities. Keep it ready to use as it is in a flour shaker, or mix up one of the following recipes. Once you start using baking soda in this way, you will be amazed at its powers for cleaning and freshening up in every room of the house.

> If you're unsure whether a cleaning product will be safe on a particular surface, try it on a small, inconspicuous area first.

Cleaning products

These simple-to-make recipes for basic natural cleaning solutions can be used all around the house. For difficult-to-clean areas, try the extra-strong versions. Make sure that you follow the guidance for use and storage.

Basic cleaning fluid

600ml/21fl oz/2½ cups warm
  water
1 tablespoon baking soda
  (bicarbonate of soda)

two squeezes of washing-up
  liquid (dish detergent)

I   Put the warm water into a large bowl and add the other
    ingredients, mixing together well.

Use and storage

Make just enough for a particular cleaning job and use it from the bowl. Alternatively, pour it into a labeled spray bottle, putting the top on only after any fizzing has stopped, and shake before each use.

BRUSHES

Clean hairbrushes, combs, toothbrushes and make-up applicators by soaking them in Basic Cleaning Fluid (see page 78) for 30 minutes, then rinsing well.

Extra-strength cleaning fluid

This is a super-charged version of the Basic Cleaning Fluid (above). It is unsuitable for waxed surfaces, or granite or other stone surfaces, because vinegar and lemon juice can cause dulling.

600ml/21fl oz/2½ cups warm water

1 tablespoon baking soda (bicarbonate of soda)

two squeezes of washing-up liquid (dish detergent)

120ml/4fl oz/½ cup white vinegar, optional

2 lemons, optional

1   Put the warm water into a large bowl and add the baking soda and washing-up liquid, mixing together well.

2   Use either vinegar or lemon, not both. If using lemon, slice the lemons in half and squeeze out the juice, straining so that there are no pips. Add the vinegar or lemon juice to the mixture. It will fizz a lot when first mixed.

Use and storage
Make just enough for a particular cleaning job and use it from the bowl. Alternatively, pour it into a labeled spray bottle, putting the top on only after any fizzing has stopped, and shake before each use.

Basic cleaning paste

This is excellent for cleaning areas of adherent grime, such as a ring around a bathtub. The amounts required depend on the size of the job. The proportions are about three parts baking soda (bicarbonate of soda) to one part water

3 tablespoons baking soda (bicarbonate of soda)
1 tablespoon water

a few drops of lemon, tea-tree or lavender essential oil, optional

1   Put the baking soda (bicarbonate of soda) into a small bowl and stir in the water to make a paste.
2   Mix in a few drops of the essential oil for fragrance, if wanted.

Use and storage
Make just enough for a particular cleaning job and use it from the bowl. If the paste starts to dry, add more water.

Extra-strength cleaning paste
Make the Basic Cleaning Paste recipe above, but using vinegar instead of water.

Use and storage
Make just enough for a particular cleaning job and use it from the bowl. If the paste starts to dry, add more water.

Cream cleaner
Make the Basic Cleaning Paste recipe above, then stir in extra water until it has the consistency of thick cream. Add a few drops of lemon, tea-tree, lavender or other essential oil for fragrance, if wanted.

Use and storage
Make enough for a particular job and use it from the bowl. Alternatively, pour it into a labeled squeezy bottle, putting the top on only after any fizzing has stopped, and shake before each use.

Scouring powder

This recipe includes borax substitute (sodium sesquicarbonate), which is available online, and salt. The borax substitute has bleaching, stain-removing, deodorizing and disinfecting qualities, whilst the salt has de-greasing and cleaning qualities.

I tablespoon baking soda
  (bicarbonate of soda)

I tablespoon borax substitute
I tablespoon table salt

1   Mix the baking soda (bicarbonate of soda), borax substitute and table salt in a bowl.
2   Apply with a scrubbing brush, a cloth or, for small hard-to-reach areas, an old toothbrush.

Use and storage
Make enough for a particular job and use it from the bowl.
Alternatively, put it into a labeled jar or plastic container.

INSECTS

Remove smears left after cleaning dead insects from
a car windscreen (windshield) by applying baking soda
(bicarbonate of soda) on a damp sponge, then rinsing
and wiping clean.

How to clean… the kitchen

You will most likely already have baking soda (bicarbonate of soda) in your kitchen cupboard, ready for use in cookery, particularly baking. Try out some of these suggestions for natural cleaning.

Hands

- Wash very soiled hands with soap, then sprinkle with baking soda (bicarbonate of soda). Rub your hands together, then rinse and dry.
- Sprinkle baking soda (bicarbonate of soda) into rubber gloves to keep them fresh and make them easy to put on.

Dirty dishes

- Add 50g/1¾oz/¼ cup of baking soda (bicarbonate of soda)and the juice of ½ a lemon to washing-up water to aid de-greasing and help loosen stuck-on food. You'll need less washing-up liquid (dish detergent) than usual.
- Store steel-wool pan scourers in baking soda (bicarbonate of soda) to prevent rust.
- Clean the kitchen sink with Extra-Strength Cleaning Fluid (see page 80) or rub all over with baking soda (bicarbonate of soda) sprinkled on a damp sponge or cloth.

Sink pipes

- Help clear a block by pouring 200g/7oz/1 cup baking soda (bicarbonate of soda) down the plughole, followed by 240ml/8fl oz/1 cup hot vinegar. Wait for 30 minutes, then flush with a kettle of just-boiled water. If necessary, use a sink plunger.

- Freshen waste pipes and prevent them from becoming blocked by pouring 100g/3½oz/½ cup of baking soda (bicarbonate of soda) down the plughole and flushing with a kettle of just-boiled water each month.

Dishwashers

- Mix 2 tablespoons of baking soda (bicarbonate of soda) with 2 tablespoons borax substitute (see page 84) to make dishwashing powder.
- Help prevent unwanted odours by filling the dishwasher-powder (or tablet) dispenser with baking soda (bicarbonate of soda) and running a rinse cycle.
- Alternatively, clean inside and out with Basic Cleaning Fluid (see page 78) or Extra-Strength Cleaning Fluid (see page 80) and wipe clean.
- Or simply sprinkle 100g/3½oz/½ cup baking soda (bicarbonate of soda) into the bottom of the dishwasher after emptying it.

Refrigerators and freezers

- Clean a refrigerator or freezer by wiping inside and out with Basic Cleaning Fluid (see page 78), then rinsing. The remaining film keeps it smelling sweet.
- Rub stained areas with Basic Cleaning Paste (see page 82), then rinse.
- Make a refrigerator or freezer smell sweet with a bowl of baking soda (bicarbonate of soda) inside. Stir it every few days and replace every 2–3 months.

Wooden chopping boards

- Spring-clean a board by sprinkling it with baking soda (bicarbonate of soda), then spraying it with white vinegar. Leave the bicarbonate-vinegar paste on for 30 minutes before rinsing with hot water.
- Deodorize a cutting board or wooden work surface that smells of garlic or onions by sprinkling some baking soda (bicarbonate of soda) on to a damp sponge, rubbing this over the board, then rinsing it clean.

SAUCEPANS

CAUTION: Do not use baking soda (bicarbonate of soda) on nonstick pans, as it can damage the surface.
Get rid of burnt-on food residues by:

- brushing or scrubbing a saucepan with baking soda (bicarbonate of soda) or Scouring Powder (see page 84). Don't scour saucepans that have an enamelled interior.
- wetting the saucepan with hot water then sprinkling on a thick layer of bicarbonate of soda. Leave overnight, then brush or scrape off the residues.
- putting 240ml/8fl oz/1 cup water into the saucepan, adding 1 tablespoon white vinegar and bringing to the boil. Add 2 tablespoons baking soda (bicarbonate of soda) and wait for the fizzing to subside, then brush or scrape off the residues.

Oven and hob

CAUTION: The Basic Cleaning Paste can mark shiny stainless steel, and baking soda (bicarbonate of soda) can darken aluminium or corrode the heating elements in an electric oven.

- Spray the oven walls with water, then spread them with a thick layer of Basic Cleaning Paste (see page 82). Leave this on for several hours, spraying with a little water every hour or so to keep the paste moist. Use a spatula, palette knife or hob scraper to remove the debris. Wipe clean.
- Deal with charred greasy food residues on an oven floor by spraying with water, sprinkling on a thick layer of baking soda (bicarbonate of soda) and spraying again. Leave for several hours, spraying every hour or so to keep the paste moist. Wipe clean.
- If necessary, clean an oven or hob with Extra-Strength Cleaning Paste (see page 82).
- Clean a greasy hob, grill or splash-back by rubbing on baking soda (bicarbonate of soda) with a damp sponge or cloth, then wiping clean.
- De-grease and clean an encrusted barbecue grill by applying Extra-Strength Cleaning Paste (see page 83), leaving for several hours, brushing with a wire brush, then wiping clean.

Microwave oven

- Clean inside a microwave oven by wiping with Basic Cleaning Fluid (see page 78).
- Alternatively, put 1 tablespoon of baking soda (bicarbonate of soda) and 240ml/8fl oz/1 cup water into

a microwaveable bowl and put this in the oven. Set the oven so the liquid boils for 3–4 minutes. Wipe the inside of the oven with a damp cloth or kitchen paper.

Sponges and cloths
Clean and deodorize sponges and cloths by soaking them in Basic Cleaning Fluid (see page 78), then rinsing and drying.

Walls, doors, work surfaces, floors and furniture
Baking soda (bicarbonate of soda) helps to clean paint, laminate, other plastic, glass, granite, other stone, composite, rubber, brick, steel, fibreglass and washable wallpaper. If using it on bare wood, be sparing with the water and dry well to avoid water marks.

- Mop or wipe floors with 100g/3½oz/½ cup baking soda (bicarbonate of soda) dissolved in a bucket of hot water.
- Wipe other surfaces with Basic Cleaning Fluid (see page 78), then rinse.
- Rub particularly soiled or stained areas with baking soda (bicarbonate of soda) on a damp sponge or cloth, then rinse.
- Banish grease or scuff marks on washable walls with baking soda (bicarbonate of soda) on a damp sponge; rinse, then wipe dry.

How to clean... the bathroom
Baking soda can be used along with other natural ingredients to create beauty treatments, as well featuring in our daily personal hygiene routine (see page 62). But it can also be used to keep the bathroom itself clean and sparkling!

- When you have a bath, add 2 tablespoons of baking soda (bicarbonate of soda) to the water. This will help to prevent a scummy ring forming around the bathtub when you drain away the water.
- Clean the bathtub, basin, taps, tiles and mirrors by using a damp cloth or sponge to apply fragranced Cream Cleaner or Basic Cleaning Paste (see pages 83 and 82). Rinse.
- Alternatively, rub with baking soda (bicarbonate of soda) sprinkled on to a damp cloth or sponge, then rinse.
- For heavier soiling or to clean glass shower screens, rub on Extra-Strength Cleaning Paste (see page 83), leave for 30 minutes, then rinse. Dry a glass shower screen with a barely damp towel.
- Clean a lavatory cistern and bowl by putting 200g/7oz/1 cup baking soda (bicarbonate of soda)into the cistern overnight, then flushing next morning. Repeat once a month.
- Clean a lavatory bowl by sprinkling baking soda (bicarbonate of soda)on to a damp scrubbing brush and scrubbing under the rim.
- Treat a stained lavatory bowl by rubbing with Extra-Strength Cleaning Paste (see page 83).
- Use an old firm-bristled toothbrush to apply Extra-Strength Cleaning Paste (see page 83) to soiled tile grouting. Leave for 30 minutes, then rinse.
- For particularly grimy grouting, mix three parts baking soda (bicarbonate of soda)with one part bleach and scrub this over the grouting with a toothbrush. Wait for 30 minutes, then rinse.

Shower head unblocker

Help prevent mineral salts in hard water blocking a shower-head.

50g/1¾oz/¼ cup baking soda
(bicarbonate of soda)

240ml/ 8fl oz/1 cup white
vinegar

1   Place the baking soda into a strong plastic bag, making sure that it doesn't have any holes.
2   Pour in the vinegar and shake to mix.
3   Tie the bag around the shower-head and leave for 30 minutes.
4   Remove, then run the water for a few seconds. (If you can remove the shower-head, simply immerse it in the above mixture for 30 minutes, then rinse.)

Shower curtain washing-boost

If a soiled or mildewed shower curtain is machine-washable, adding baking soda and vinegar to the machine cycle will get it sparkling clean again.

200g/7oz/1 cup baking soda (bicarbonate of soda)

washing powder or liquid detergent
120ml/4fl oz/½ cup of white vinegar

1   Put the shower curtain in the washing machine along with a large bath towel.
2   Add the baking soda (bicarbonate of soda) to the washing powder or liquid detergent when adding to the machine.
3   Wash the shower curtain and towel on a low-temperature setting.
4   During the rinse cycle, adding the white vinegar to the fabric-softener dispenser. Don't spin fast, or the curtain could become permanently creased.
5   Hang up to dry.

- Clean a non-machine-washable shower curtain by soaking it for 30 minutes in a bath of warm water containing about 150g/5½oz/¾ cup bicarbonate of soda. Rinse and drip-dry.

FIRES

If you don't have a fire extinguisher or a fire blanket at the ready, but you do have a large amount of baking soda (bicarbonate of soda) to hand, put out a small grease or oil fire, or an electrical fire, by throwing baking soda (bicarbonate of soda) over it. (Water is unsafe for either sort of fire). But don't use baking soda (bicarbonate of soda) on a deep-fat-fryer fire, as it could make the flaming grease splatter. Also, take no risks and, if necessary, get yourself and others out of the house and make sure that someone calls the fire service.

Sprinkle baking soda (bicarbonate of soda) on to floors or worktops or in cupboards to repel unwanted insects.

How to clean... baby and child equipment and toys

- Dip children's dirty washable toys into Basic Cleaning Fluid (see page 78), or use a cloth to wipe them with this. Rinse and dry.
- Wash a plastic paddling pool and remove any mildew with Basic Cleaning Fluid (see page 78).
- Clean high-chairs, car-seats, buggies (strollers) and plastic mattress protectors by sprinkling baking soda (bicarbonate of soda) on to a damp sponge, rubbing with this, then wiping with a clean sponge several times.
- Remove milk residues from a baby's bottles, teats (nipples) and bottle brushes by soaking them in Basic Cleaning Fluid (see page 78). Rinse, then sterilize as usual.

How to clean... fruits and vegetables
Many people wash fruits and vegetables before eating them to get rid of dirt, pesticide traces and micro-organisms. You could just use water, but a baking soda (bicarbonate of soda) solution is better.

- Wash fruits and vegetables in a solution of 1 teaspoon baking soda (bicarbonate of soda) dissolved in a bowl of water, then rinse.
- Shake a little baking soda (bicarbonate of soda) on to a wet vegetable brush and gently scrub firm fruits and vegetables.
- Clean soft fruits with a damp sponge sprinkled with baking soda (bicarbonate of soda).

PLANT CARE

- Spray plant foliage affected by mildew fungi with Basic Cleaning Fluid (see page 78) in the evening.
- To treat plant foliage affected by black-spot fungi, add 1 teaspoon of cooking oil to a bottle of Basic Cleaning Fluid (see page 78) and spray in the evening.
- Clean vases inside by filling with hot water and adding 2 tablespoons of baking soda (bicarbonate of soda). Leave for 1 hour, then rinse.

How to clean... metal

Baking soda (bicarbonate of soda) can help to clean silver, chrome and copper. It has even been used to clean the copper Statue of Liberty in New York.

Do not, however, use it on aluminium, as it would remove the thin protective coating of aluminium oxide. Bare aluminium reacts to acid so would soon look patchy if touched with sweaty hands or exposed to city air.

Scrub a silver item with an old toothbrush and some Basic Cleaning Paste (see page 82). Rinse with warm water, dry with kitchen paper, then polish with a soft cloth.

- Put tarnished silver on aluminium foil in a bowl of warm water containing 1 teaspoon of baking soda (bicarbonate of soda). (Or put the silver item into warm water in an aluminium container). Wait 5–15 minutes, then remove, rinse, dry with kitchen paper and polish with a soft cloth. Silver reacts with oxygen and sulphur gases in the air to form a tarnish containing silver sulphide. In turn, aluminium reacts with silver sulphide to form aluminium sulphide, leaving sparkly bright pure silver.
- Clean chrome on car bumpers (fenders) and hubcaps, or on a bicycle, by rubbing baking soda (bicarbonate of soda) over them with a damp sponge. Rinse, then polish with a soft dry cloth.
- Make stainless steel shine by rubbing on baking soda (bicarbonate of soda)with a damp sponge, then rinsing and drying.
- Clean brass or copper objects by rubbing with baking soda (bicarbonate of soda) sprinkled on to half a lemon. Rinse and dry.

- De-grime gold jewellery by putting it into a bowl, sprinkling it with baking soda (bicarbonate of soda), then pouring white vinegar over it. Rinse and dry. However, don't do this if the jewellery contains pearls or if gemstones have been glued in place rather than captured in metal 'claws'.

RUST REMOVING

Help remove rust from metal by applying Basic Cleaning Paste (see page 82) with a damp cloth. Scrub lightly with a piece of aluminium foil, rinse and dry with kitchen paper.

Stain removing

For stains on clothing, see 'Laundering' (page 101).

- Clean fruit drink or fruit juice stains from kitchen work surfaces or other washable surfaces by spraying them with water, then sprinkling them with baking soda (bicarbonate of soda). Leave for 30 minutes, then wipe clean.
- Remove crayon marks on a painted or papered wall by sprinkling baking soda (bicarbonate of soda) on to a damp sponge, rubbing the wall very gently, then wiping clean.
- Eradicate water spots on wooden floors by dabbing with a sponge or cloth dampened with Basic Cleaning Fluid (see page 78). Wipe clean and repeat several times to remove all traces of baking soda (bicarbonate of soda). Dry well. Don't wet the wood too much, as this could simply make more water spots!
- Deal with a stained laminate (or other plastic) or marble worktop or other surface by rubbing on some Basic Cleaning Paste (see page 82), then rinsing.
- Clean a stained vacuum flask or one that you haven't used for some time by putting 1–2 teaspoons of baking soda (bicarbonate of soda) into the flask and filling it with hot water. Leave for 30 minutes, then rinse well.
- Remove wine, grease and certain other stains from carpet by lightly wetting the stains, then sprinkling them with baking soda (bicarbonate of soda). Leave to dry, then vacuum up the residue.
- Apply Extra-Strength Cleaning Paste (see page 83) to ink stains on hard floors, then rinse and dry.
- Clean brown staining on the base of your iron by unplugging and cooling it first, then rubbing with Basic Cleaning Paste.

Get rid of tannin stains from tea and coffee by:

- using a damp sponge to rub baking soda (bicarbonate of soda) on to cups and mugs, leaving for 30 minutes, then rinsing.
- filling cups and mugs with warm water and adding ½ teaspoon of baking soda (bicarbonate of soda). Leave for 30 minutes, then rinse.
- filling a coffee pot or teapot with hot water and adding 2 teaspoons of baking soda (bicarbonate of soda) and 2 teaspoons of white vinegar. Leave for 30 minutes, then rinse.
- filling a glass and metal (but not aluminium) cafetière with hot water, stirring in 1 teaspoon of baking soda (bicarbonate of soda)and 1 teaspoon of white vinegar, and leaving it to soak for 30 minutes before rinsing.

Laundering

Baking soda (bicarbonate of soda) makes an excellent stain remover and deodorizer – it is the perfect addition to your laundry supplies.

- Keep your laundry basket fresh by sprinkling a little baking soda (bicarbonate of soda) into it each day.
- Clean your washing machine drum, and inside the door, with Basic Cleaning Fluid or, for stubborn marks, Basic Cleaning Paste (see pages 78 and 82).
- Deodorize your washing machine drum, and inside the door, by wiping with Basic Cleaning Fluid (see page 78).
- Alternatively, clean the washing machine by putting 50g/1¾oz/ ¼ cup of baking soda (bicarbonate of soda) into the washing-powder dispenser and 240ml/8fl oz/¼ cup of white vinegar into the fabric-softener dispenser before running the machine on a short cycle.
- Add 100g/3½oz/½ cup of baking soda (bicarbonate of soda) along with your usual amount of liquid washing detergent to the washing machine or hand-wash bowl for more effective washing power. This also helps shift many sorts of stain.
- Help to whiten white clothes by adding 100g/3½oz/½ cup of baking soda (bicarbonate of soda)to the washing-powder dispenser, or, if washing by hand, to the final rinse water.
- Alternatively, add 50g/1¾oz/¼ cup of baking soda (bicarbonate of soda) to a basin of cold water, immerse the clothing and soak overnight. Next morning, wash as usual.
- For greater whitening action, add the juice of a lemon and 50g/1¾oz/¼ cup of baking soda (bicarbonate of soda) to a basin of cold water. Soak the clothing overnight and wash it next morning.

- Alternatively, boost the performance of bleach by adding 100g/3½oz/½ cup of baking soda (bicarbonate of soda) and 240ml/4fl oz/½ cup of bleach to a bowl of water.
- Whiten cloth nappies (diapers) by adding 100g/3½oz/½ cup of baking soda (bicarbonate of soda) to the washing-powder dispenser, or along with the washing powder if hand-washing.
- Use baking soda (bicarbonate of soda) to make chlorine bleach more effective: add 100g/3½oz/½ cup along with the usual amount of bleach.
- Deodorize soiled cloth nappies (diapers) by putting 50g/1¾oz/ ¼ cup of baking soda (bicarbonate of soda) into a bucket of cold water and soaking them overnight. Next morning, wash as usual.
- If clothing is stained with something acidic (such as fruit juice or tomato sauce), pre-treating it with baking soda (bicarbonate of soda) before washing should prevent the acid eating into the fabric; it should also loosen the stain. Sprinkle with baking soda (bicarbonate of soda), spray with water then leave for 30 minutes before washing. This is also effective for acidic sweat, vomit and urine stains.
- Remove a blood stain by putting 100g/3½oz/½ cup of baking soda (bicarbonate of soda) and 120ml/4fl oz/½ cup of white vinegar into a bowl of cold water and soaking the item in this mixture overnight. Wash as normal next day.
- Get rid of grease on clothing by applying a paste of baking soda (bicarbonate of soda) and water, leaving for 30 minutes then adding 100g/3½oz/½ cup of baking soda (bicarbonate of soda)to the washing machine (or a bowl if hand-washing) along with the liquid detergent. Run your usual cycle.

- Or make a paste from two parts of baking soda (bicarbonate of soda), one part of cream of tartar and a little water and rub this on a grease mark before washing.
- Rub a tar stain with Basic Cleaning Paste (see page 82) then wash it with baking soda (bicarbonate of soda) and water.
- Remove a rust stain from clothing by soaking it in lemon juice then sprinkling with a thick layer of baking soda (bicarbonate of soda). Leave overnight, then rinse and wash.
- Try eliminating a mildew smell from fabric by soaking it in Basic Cleaning Fluid (see page 78) overnight, then washing.

Fabric softener (conditioner)

200g/7oz/1 cup baking soda
(bicarbonate of soda)
240ml/8fl oz/1 cup vinegar

480ml/16fl oz/2 cups water
3–4 drops lemon, lavender or
rose essential oil, optional

1   Put the baking soda (bicarbonate of soda), vinegar and water
    into a bottle large enough to accommodate the effervescence
    produced when baking soda (bicarbonate of soda) mixes with
    vinegar.
2   Add the essential oil, if using, and mix well.
3   Add 60ml/2fl oz/¼ cup of this mixture to your washing
    machine's fabric-softener dispenser when you do a wash, or
    put it into the final rinse water if handwashing. Baking soda
    (bicarbonate of soda) helps to make towels soft and fluffy.

Deodorizing

Baking soda (bicarbonate of soda) neutralizes unpleasant smells. It acts against odours from acidic substances (such as in sweat, urine or vomit) and alkaline ones (such as ammonia from wet nappies/diapers).

- Prevent unpleasant smells in a larder or store cupboard by keeping a small open bowl of baking soda (bicarbonate of soda) in it. Stir every few days and replace every 2–3 months.
- Eliminate stale smells from plastic bowls or food containers by filling them with hot water and stirring in 1 tablespoon of baking soda (bicarbonate of soda). Soak for 30 minutes, then rinse.
- If the smell persists, repeat, adding 1 tablespoon of vinegar and a few drops of washing-up liquid (dish detergent) along with the baking soda (bicarbonate of soda).
- Add a small handful of baking soda (bicarbonate of soda) to keep a kitchen-rubbish (garbage) container smelling sweet.
- Prevent unpleasant smells from your waste-disposal unit (garbage-disposer) by each week pouring 2 tablespoons of baking soda (bicarbonate of soda) and 1 tablespoon of white vinegar into it and running hot water from the tap as you operate the disposer.
- Make a stored blanket smell sweeter by shaking baking soda (bicarbonate of soda) over it, then rolling it up. Leave overnight, then shake it next morning and tumble it in the tumble drier set to cold.
- Deodorize carpets and rugs by shaking baking soda (bicarbonate of soda) all over them, waiting at least 30 minutes, then vacuuming.

- After cleaning spilt drink or food from a carpet, sprinkle with baking soda (bicarbonate of soda), wait 30 minutes, then vacuum. This makes an unpleasant smell less likely to linger.
- Deodorize the carpet in your car by sprinkling it with baking soda (bicarbonate of soda), leaving for at least 30 minutes, then vacuuming.
- Leave a small pot of baking soda (bicarbonate of soda) in each room to act as an air freshener by neutralizing any unwanted odour. Commercial air fresheners mostly act by producing a masking scent.
- Home-make a fragranced air freshener by adding a few drops of lemon, geranium, lavender, neroli, rose or other essential oil to a small pot of baking soda (bicarbonate of soda).
- Neutralize a sour odour from cleaned-up human or pet vomit stains by sprinkling generously with baking soda (bicarbonate of soda). Leave for several hours, then vacuum.
- Sprinkle baking soda (bicarbonate of soda) into smelly shoes, boots or trainers, leave overnight and then, next morning, tap out the surplus. (Note that doing this with leather shoes could stiffen the leather.)
- Keep a wardrobe (closet) smelling sweet by putting an open bowl of baking soda (bicarbonate of soda) inside. Add a few drops of lemon, geranium, lavender, neroli, rose or other essential oil for special fragrance.
- Alternatively, use scraps of fabric to make little bags which you can fill with baking soda (bicarbonate of soda) and, perhaps, some fragrant essential oil, tie up with string or ribbon, and keep inside a wardrobe or drawer.

- Sprinkle baking soda (bicarbonate of soda) into garment storage bags to prevent musty smells.
- Freshen stuffed toys by sprinkling with baking soda (bicarbonate of soda). Wait for 30 minutes, then brush off.
- If there's a smoker in your home, put baking soda (bicarbonate of soda) into the ashtrays to combat the tobacco smell.
- Sprinkle tents, waterproofs and other camping gear with baking soda (bicarbonate of soda) before storing.
- Rid a vacuum flask of stale smells by filling it with hot water and adding 2 teaspoons of baking soda (bicarbonate of soda). Soak for 30 minutes, then rinse.
- Help prevent odour from a pet's litter tray by putting a thick layer of baking soda (bicarbonate of soda) on the bottom of the tray before adding the litter.
- Also, sprinkle baking soda (bicarbonate of soda) over a cat litter tray to help neutralize unpleasant smells.
- To remove the wet-dog smell from a damp dog's coat, sprinkle with baking soda (bicarbonate of soda), wait 30 minutes, then brush it out.
- Make a dog's or cat's bedding smell better by sprinkling it with baking soda (bicarbonate of soda), leaving it for 1 hour, then vacuuming.

INDEX